Balboa Press books may be ordered through booksellers or by contacting:

Balboa Press
A Division of Hay House
1663 Liberty Drive
Bloomington, IN 47403
www.balboapress.com.au
AU TFN: 1 800 844 925 (Toll Free inside Australia)
AU Local: 0283 107 086 (+61 2 8310 7086 from outside Australia)

ISBN: 978-1-5043-2374-1 (sc)
ISBN: 978-1-5043-2375-8 (e)

Print information available on the last page.

Balboa Press rev. date: 12/02/2020

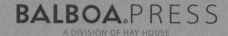

BALBOAPRESS
A DIVISION OF HAY HOUSE

How I Cured My Chronic Muscle Inflammation
In Just 29 Days!

By Kathrin M Allen

7 Years Pain Maintenance

I was lying on the massage table when my masseur pushed down on my spine, grunted, and said 'Wow! Your back's like concrete.' 'It's like your muscles are clinging to your skeleton for dear life!'

I knew what he meant. Try to imagine a rubber-band ball wound so tight it bounces when dropped.

For 7 years I had been visiting chiropractors, physiotherapists, Pilates instructors and masseurs. I found without these sessions I couldn't turn my head. My shoulders and neck crunched. And my back, glutes, and quadriceps were so tight they'd pull me out of alignment.

My muscles were constantly tense, and the burning sensation persisted regardless of treatment. I'd tried everything, even acupuncture, but I only ever experienced momentary relief.

Enough was enough.

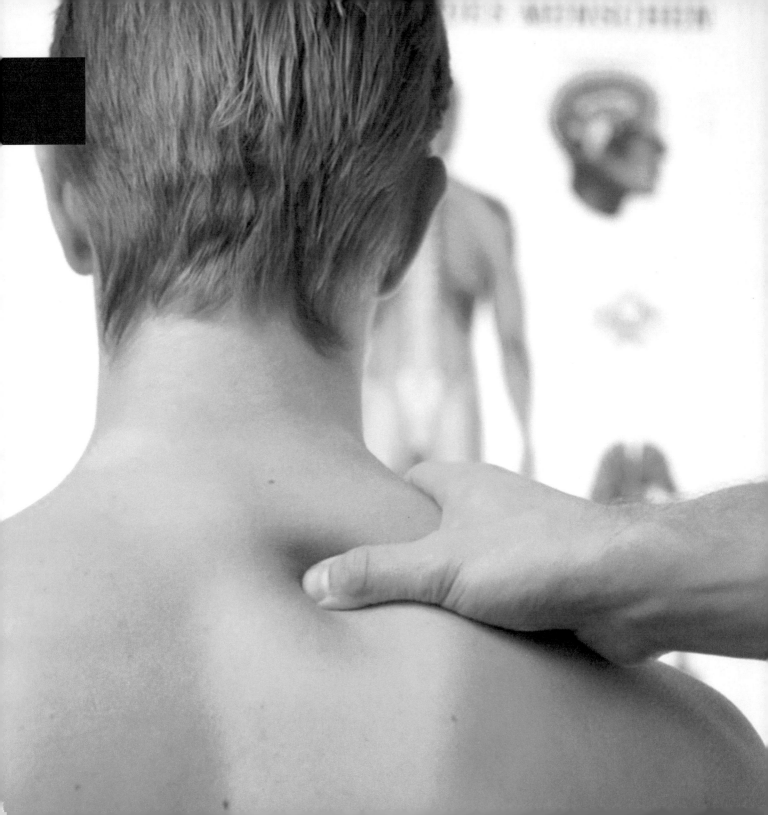

I decided to take accountability for my own healing, and embarked on a journey over the next 12 months.

My goal, to discover the physical, mental, and spiritual support systems that would enable me to live my best life.

Today, as I write this, I am 47 and living a happy, healthy, completely pain & drug free existence.

Here is my story on how I cured my chronic muscle inflammation in just 29 days.

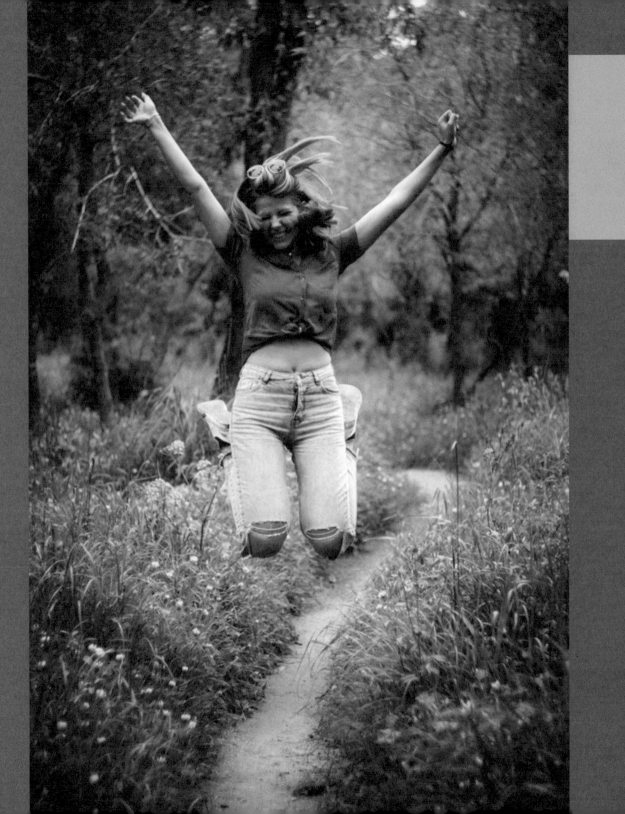

Why Drug Free?

As a young child I used to watch my Grandma take her egg cup and fill it with her pills at breakfast. Now I watch my Father work his way through 32 pharmaceutical tablets a day. This created in me an aversion to drugs, and I am adamant I will not medicate myself in this way.

In todays world we are encouraged to rely on pharmaceutical drugs, and I want to commend my Physiotherapists, and Chiropractors, for never recommending a pharmaceutical drug to manage my inflammation.

Reliance on pharmaceutical products and pricey health specialists, is not part of my goal.

And so I began exploring different forms of movement, and it was here that I discovered Qi Gong.

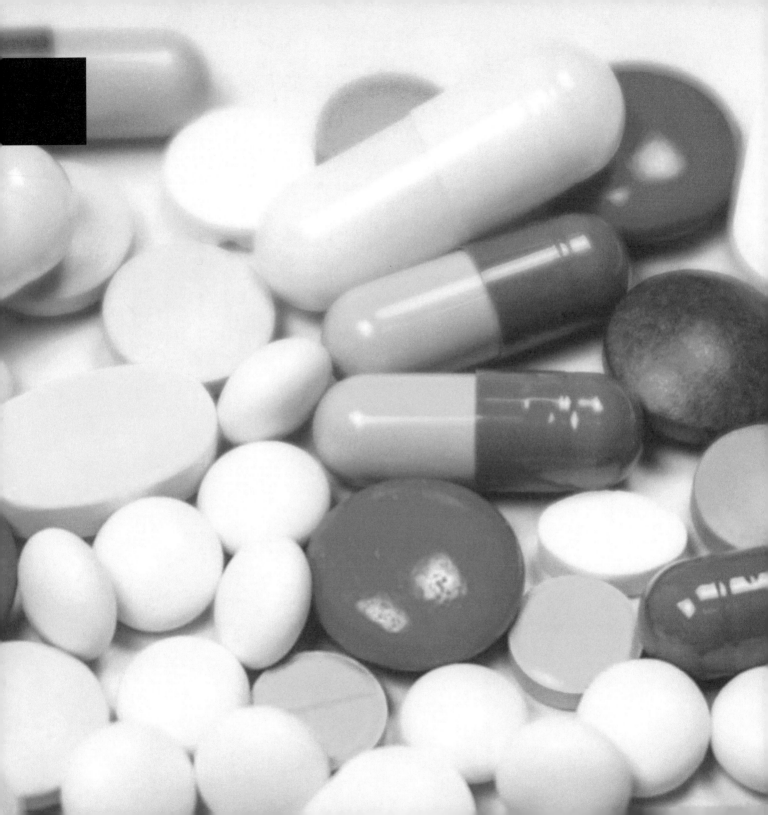

Movement

Qigong is a system of coordinated body-postures, movements, breathing, and meditation, used for the purposes of health, spirituality, and martial-arts training.

In mastering this practice, I found that my flexibility and strength improved, and I was less prone to lower back pain.

My body was now moving in ways it had not been able to for years. Inspired by this I joined my local gym.

Working with my personal trainer we tailored a program that incorporated key stretches and weight training to complement my Qi Gong.

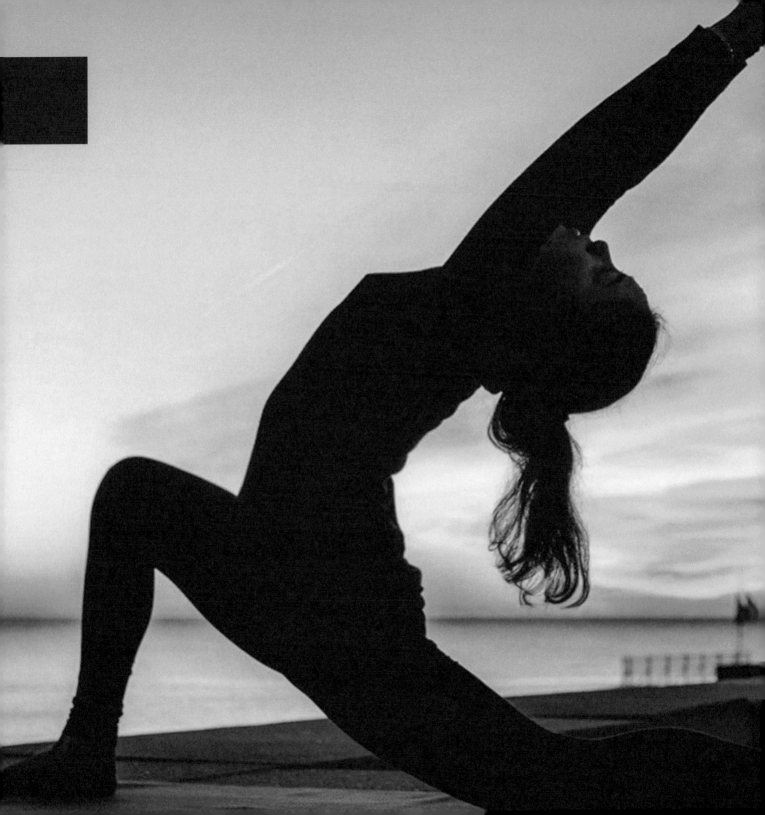

In addition to my training I began attending Yin Yoga classes.

Yin Yoga is a slow-paced exercise with asanas that are held longer, and go deeper, than in other yoga styles.

I adored every minute of Yin Yoga. It felt like 1 hour of nurturing indulgence.

However, as euphoric as Yin Yoga left me feeling, it was making zero difference to my inflammation.

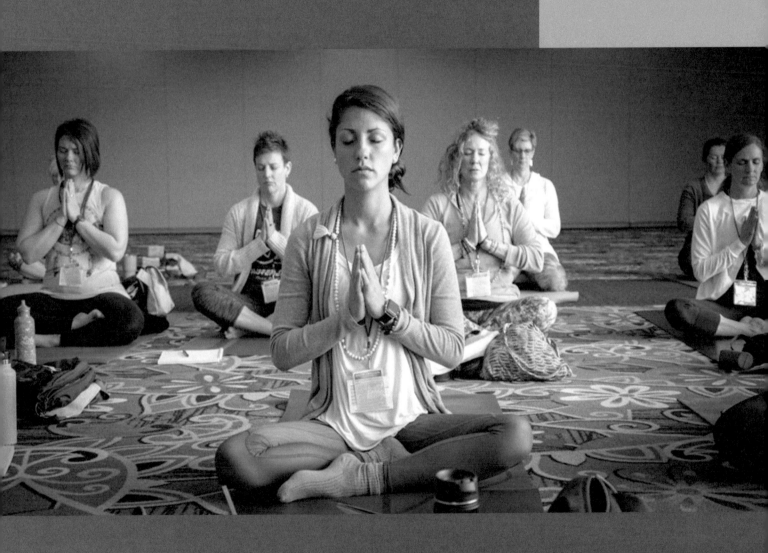

Diet – The Cure!

Now that I was taking better care of myself physically, I became curious about wholefoods, herbs, and spices.

Fascinated with the idea of Food as Medicine I learned as much as I could. Cook books were bought by the dozen and my kitchen windowsill filled up with a variety of potted herbs.

I also devoured videos on Shaman practices, and I was watching episode 5 of the Sacred Science docu-series 'Remedy' when I had an epiphany!

In this episode Paul Bergner, Director of the North American Institute of Medical Herbalism, suggests symptoms are often the result of a food intolerance rather than a disease.

Light bulb moment! Maybe my diet is causing my inflammation?

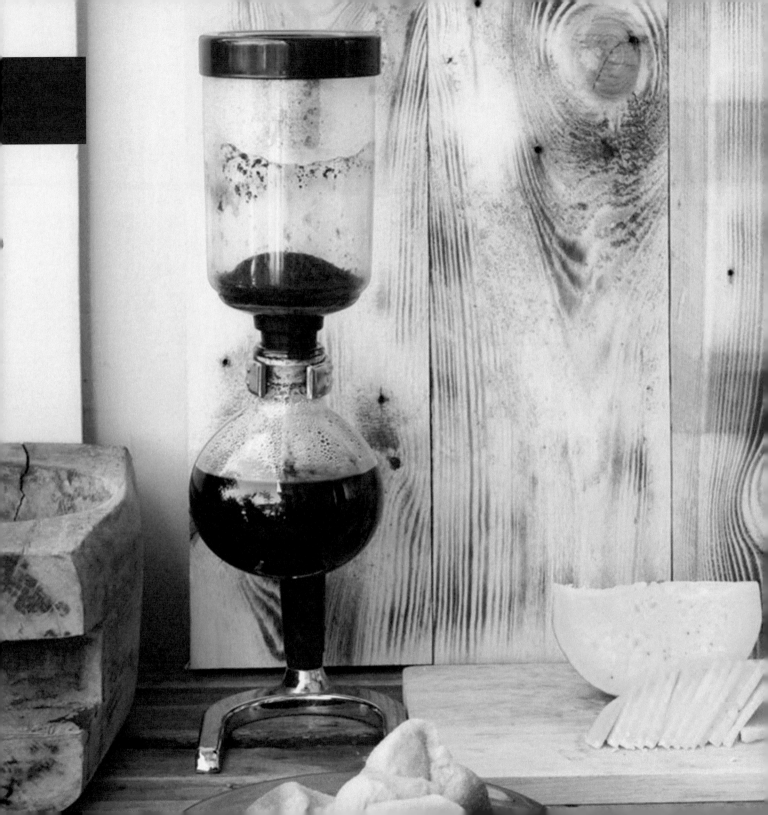

Without thinking too hard I knew I indulged in too much:

1. Coffee – Double shots
2. Cheese – Daily snack

My research told me that giving up these two items would decrease insomnia, nervousness, restlessness, increased heart and breathing rate, as well as lower my levels of saturated fats and salt, and <u>acid</u>.

Having read that high acid levels cause the body to leach alkaline from our bones to restore it's balance, I became convinced my acid levels were the cause of my chronic inflammation.

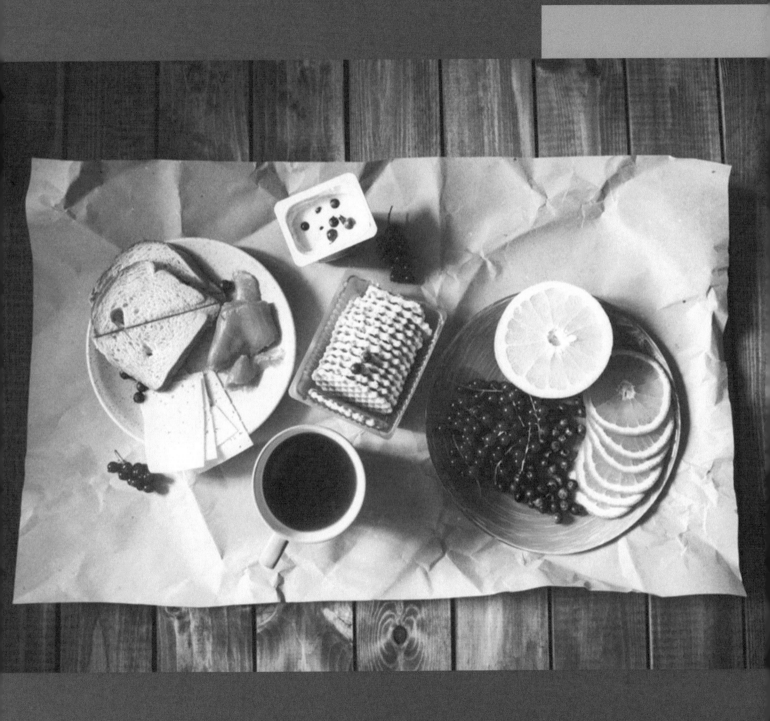

The Experiment

I made a commitment to quit coffee and cheese for a period of 30 days. During this experiment I swapped cow milk for Oat milk. Coffee for Green Tea. And I didn't eat any cheese.

In just **29 days**, I was excited to record in my journal, that I no longer felt even a hint of the constant pain I had been living with for the past 7 years.

In under one month, I had become **inflammation free!** I was stunned. My shoulders and neck now moved freely. My muscle groups felt limber.

Do you want to know the craziest thing? I don't miss the coffee at all!

And, I still eat cheese, in moderation, with no signs of my inflammation returning. This experiment was conducted in 2018, and to this day I remain inflammation free.

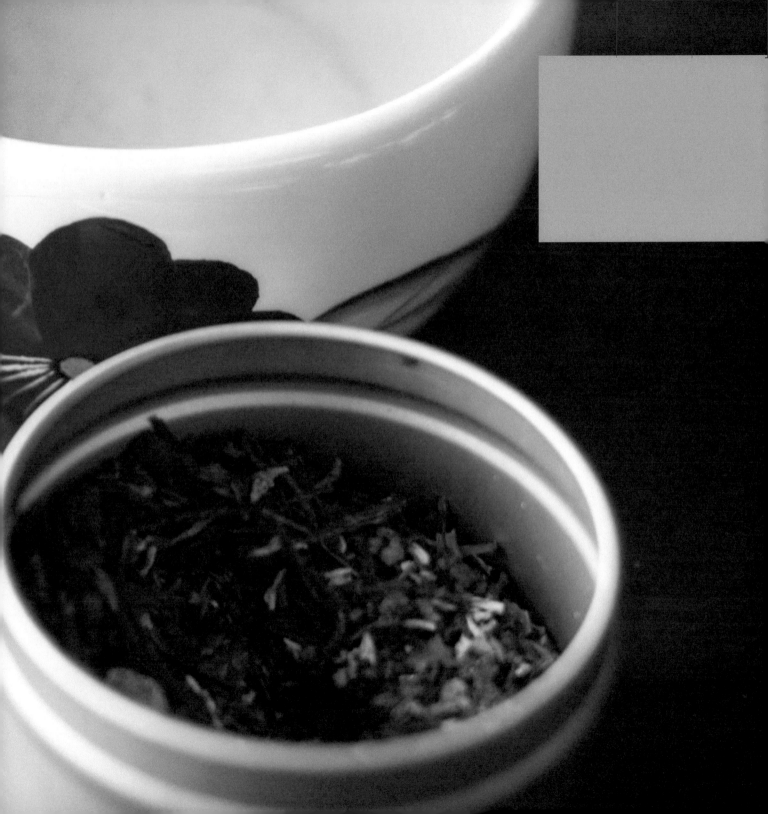

These 2 simple changes to my diet have set me free from a life of constant pain.

Allowing me to live a life I enjoy in its fullest.

I hope in telling my story, you too will discover the physical, mental, and spiritual support systems that enable you to live your best life.

Looking for more ways to boost your health naturally? Discover my 5 Go To Herbs for Anxiety Relief & Immune System Support

Kathrin M Allen is a Cartoonist, Copywriter, Content Writer & Blogger https://www.kathrinmallen.com.au/

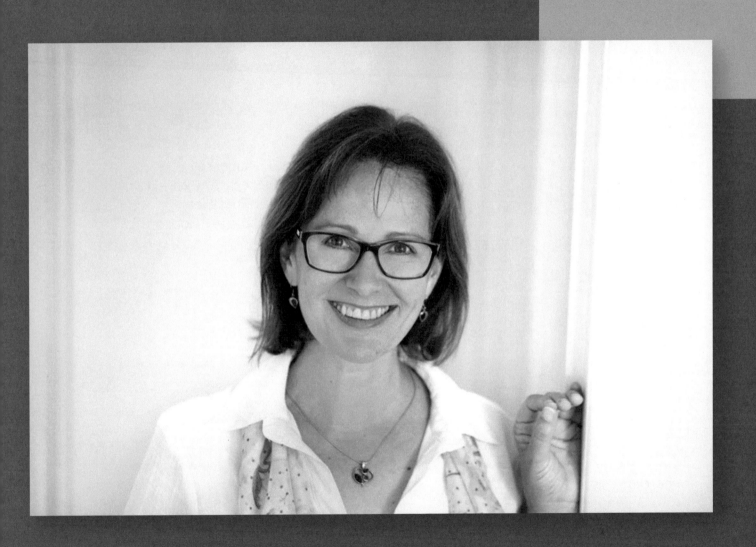

Resources	Reference Type	Template
Nick Polizzi's 'Remedy - Ancient Medicine for Modern Illness' Docu-Series	Website	Retrieved from: https://remedy.thesacredscience.com/register-g
QiGong Flow Form	Website	Retrieved from: https://www.satoriqigong.com/program.php
Matching your Herbs to Yourself, Not Your Ailment	Book	De la Foret, R., (2017). Alchemy of Herbs – Transform Everday Ingredients Into Foods & Remedies That Heal. United States of America, Hay House Inc.
Photo 1 – Man in Physiotherapists Office	Website	Photo by Jesper Aggergaard on Unsplash
Photo 2 – Girl jumping for joy	Website	Photo by Dmitry Shamis on Unsplash
Photo 3 - Pills	Website	Photo by freestocks on Unsplash
Photo 4 – Qi Gong Pose	Website	Photo by kike vega on Unsplash
Photo 5 – Yoga Room	Website	Photo by Erik Brolin on Unsplash
Photo 6 – Coffee, rolls & cheese	Website	Photo by Lawrence Aritao on Unsplash
Photo 7 – Cheese Platter	Website	Photo by Anastasia Zhenina on Unsplash
Photo 8 – Green Tea background	Website	Photo by Sheelah Brennan on Unsplash

NOTES

NOTES

NOTES

NOTES

NOTES

NOTES

_____

_____

_____

_____

_____

_____

_____

_____

_____

_____

_____

NOTES

NOTES

NOTES

NOTES

Printed in the United States
By Bookmasters